Quick Immune System Boosting Recipes Cookbook

Recipes And Preparation Instructions To Help You Recover And Boost Your Immune System.

By

Frank L. Daugherty

The trademarks that are used are without any consent, and the publication of the trademark is without permission or backing by the trademark owner. All trademarks and brands within this book are for clarifying purposes only and are owned by the owners themselves, not affiliated with this document.

Table of Contents

Introduction

Autoimmune disorders allow healthy cells in the body to be targeted by the immune response. Autoimmune infection can cause the intestinal tract covering, contributing to increased gut microbiota or "leaky gut." This enables entry into the bloodstream of materials and waste materials, causing inflammation. In the people with an autoimmune disease, the autoimmune treatment diet, or AIP diet, focuses on curing the stomach by removing foods that induce symptoms of inflammation. As it excludes many of the same ingredients, such as legumes, the AIP diet is close to the Paleo diet strategy. However, it is more conservative than the Paleo diet and therefore does not permit many of the items typically found in the Paleo diet to be eaten.

The AIP diet could be dated directly to scientist Dr. Loren Cordain, who noticed that in those with an autoimmune disorder, certain foods permitted on the diet plan, such as nuts, beans, eggs, dairy products, and nightshade veggies, could cause symptoms. In 2010, in his book, "The Paleo Cure", senior research biochemist and wellness specialist Robb Wolf talked about the AIP diet. He described it as a 1-month diet where some foods are removed and then gradually reintroduced back into the diet to test tolerance. Dr. Sarah Ballantyne started posting on her blog, "The Paleo Mother," about the AIP diet soon afterward. She is regarded as one of the foremost authorities on both the autoimmune protocol and the complicated relationship between diet and autoimmunity.

To everyone, however, the AIP diet might not be truly helpful. However, the autoimmune protocol plan may be the secret to keeping your pain under control. While by having the foods that cause you to suffer from an autoimmune disorder, you will feel that your symptoms are influenced by the foods you consume.

This book, "AIP Diet Cookbook" will provide you with all the related information you need to understand about the autoimmune disease and introduce the AIP diet into your lifestyle.

The first chapter of this book will provide you the general information about autoimmune disease and how it affects a person. Moreover, it will give you an understanding of the autoimmune diet and the benefits of this diet. In the second chapter, you will learn what to eat and what to avoid while starting your AIP diet plan. In the third chapter, you will learn some tasty recipes to prepare breakfast and brunch, including soups and salads. The fourth chapter is about lunch and dinner recipes having vegetarian meal recipes, poultry, meat, and seafood recipes of all types. In the fifth chapter, snacks, drinks, sauces, sweets, and dessert recipes have been described to make your daily meal more special with these side dishes. Finally, a conclusion is given to make you realize how vital the AIP diet is for you regardless of whether you have the disease or not. This diet will improve your health and lower the risks of getting an autoimmune disease. Start reading this book and follow simple strategies to plan your meals with the autoimmune diet protocol meal plan.

Chapter 1: Lunch and Dinner Recipes

1.1 Vegetarian Meals for Lunch and Dinner

Harissa Portobello Mushroom Tacos

Cooking Time: 30 minutes

Serving Size: 6

Calories: 111

Ingredients:

Portobello Mushrooms

- pinch of salt
- 1 tablespoon (chopped) cilantro
- 1-pound Portobello mushrooms
- ¼ cup spicy harissa
- 2 tablespoons (chopped) red onion
- 1 ½ to 2 tablespoons lemon or lime juice
- 1 teaspoon onion powder
- 6 collard green leaves

Guacamole

- 3 tablespoons olive oil (divided)
- 1 teaspoon ground cumin
- 2 medium ripe avocados
- 2 tablespoons (chopped) tomatoes

Optional Toppings

- Cilantro (Chopped)
- cashew cream
- (Chopped) tomatoes

Method:

1. Wash and drain mushrooms.

2. Take a bowl and mix harissa with spices.
3. Coat mushrooms with harissa mixture and marinate for 15 minutes on room temperature.
4. Prepare guacamole by mashing avocados and tomatoes.
5. Add olive oil and ground cumin, lemon juice, and cilantro.
6. Wash and drain green leaves.
7. Take a skillet and add 1 tablespoon olive oil.
8. Add mushrooms and fry for 5 minutes.
9. When soft and brown, remove and set aside.
10. Take green leaves and add Portobello.
11. Add guacamole and remaining ingredients. Serve hot with salad.

Paleo Vegan Zucchini Cauliflower Fritters

Cooking Time: 10 minutes

Serving Size: 8

Calories: 54

Ingredients:

Original version

- 2 large eggs
- ½ teaspoon of sea salt
- ½ head cauliflower 3 cups, (chopped)
- ¼ cup coconut flour
- 2 medium zucchinis
- ¼ teaspoon black pepper

Egg-Free version

- ½ teaspoon of sea salt
- ¼ teaspoon black pepper
- 2 medium zucchinis
- ¼ cup all-purpose flour
- ½ head cauliflower 3 cups, (chopped)

Method:

1. In a food processor or high-speed blender, grate the zucchini.
2. For about 5 minutes, steam the cauliflower until just fork tender. In the food processor, add the cauliflower and process until it is split down into tiny chunks. Do not over-process it, or it is going to become a mess.
3. Squeeze as much moisture as possible out of the grated vegetables using a dishtowel or nuts milk bottle.
4. Put the flour of your selection, egg, salt, pepper, and any other spices you want in a pan. Whisk them.
5. Form into tiny patties or burgers.
6. In a large pan, heat 2 teaspoons of coconut oil.
7. Add four burgers to the pan and cook 2-3 minutes on either side on medium heat. For the second half of the burgers, repeat the same procedure.
8. Serve with the chosen dipping sauce or low-calorie burger bun.

Caramelized Onion Spaghetti Squash

Cooking Time: 35 minutes

Serving Size: 2

Calories: 628

Ingredients:

- Salt and pepper to taste
- a sprinkle of parmesan cheese
- ¼ cup olive oil
- 1 cup kale
- 3 lb. spaghetti squash
- 2 tablespoon butter
- 2 medium yellow onions (peeled + sliced)
- 1 ½ cup mushrooms

- ¼ teaspoon rosemary

Method:

1. Halve the squash, extract the seeds, and put them on the baking sheet.
2. On all sides of the squash, rub 2 tablespoons of olive oil and then put it face down in the baking tray.
3. Melt butter and last 2 tablespoons oil over medium-high in a broad skillet when roasting squash.
4. Add the onions, stirring regularly, to the skillet. Add the mushrooms after five minutes.
5. The onions will start caramelizing after 10 minutes. Apply an extra tablespoon of oil if they appear like they are burning at all.
6. Apply the kale to the pan and keep stirring until the onions turn a perfect golden-brown color.
7. Remove the squash from the oven after 55 minutes and give 5 minutes to it to cool down.
8. Use a spoon to extract "spaghetti" from the squash and put it in a skillet until it is slightly cool. Place rosemary, seasoning, and stir it together.

Sweet Potato Toast

Cooking Time: 20 minutes

Serving Size: 4

Calories: 80

Ingredients:

- 1 avocado
- 1 cup tuna
- 1 cup mayonnaise
- 3 sweet potatoes
- 1 red onion
- 1 cup relish
- salt and pepper to taste

- 1 lemon zest
- 1 tablespoon almond butter
- 1 banana slices
- ½ tablespoon cinnamon

Method:

1. Round the sweet potatoes into ¼ inch pieces lengthwise.
2. Attach the toaster on high heat and bake.
3. Remove the avocado layer and slice it.
4. Apply the salt, some lemon zest, and pepper to the toast.
5. Spread the toast with some almond butter and add the sliced banana and a little cinnamon.
6. To the tiny can of tuna, add 1 tablespoon of sliced red onion, 1 tablespoon of mayonnaise, and 2 tablespoons of relish.
7. Scoop on the toast with tuna.

Soft Veggie Tacos with Green Tortillas

Cooking Time: 50 minutes

Serving Size: 6

Calories: 187.8

Ingredients:

For the soft green tortillas

- ½ teaspoon AIP baking powder
- ½ cup (packed) fresh cilantro
- ⅔ cup lukewarm water
- 1 cup cassava flour
- 1 tablespoon coconut flour
- 3 tablespoons olive oil
- ½ teaspoon apple cider vinegar
- ¾ teaspoon fine sea salt

For the green sauce

- 1 cup (packed) fresh cilantro

- 1½ tablespoons lime juice
- ½ teaspoon of sea salt
- 1 cup full-fat coconut milk

To assemble the tacos

- ½ cucumber (thinly sliced)
- 2 avocados (thinly sliced)
- Fresh cilantro, for garnish
- 2 cups baby arugula
- 3 small (firm) peaches

Method:

1. Combine the coconut flour, salt, cassava flour, and baking powder in a dish to make the tortillas. Stir well.
2. In a blender, add hot water, vegetable oil, cider, and cilantro and process until thoroughly combined, for about thirty seconds.
3. To dry the ingredients, add the liquid mixture and work with a spatula to loosely blend.
4. End with your palms until smooth dough shapes by kneading a few times.
5. Divide half of the dough, then split each half into three different parts, making small balls.
6. Roll it out every ball to form a small, circular circle of about six inches in length between two sheets of baking parchment.
7. For each tortilla, insert a strip of parchment paper, so they do not adhere.
8. Over a medium-high fire, prepare a non-stick pan.
9. Heat each tortilla, open, for about two min, until the underside shows little brown spots.
10. Turn and heat on the other side for an extra 1 to 2 minutes.
11. Mix fresh cilantro, coconut milk, lemon juice, and sea salt in a blender to make a green Chile sauce and mix

well until creamy, for about 30 seconds. Refrigerate until it is required.

12. Divide the cucumber, arugula, avocados, and peaches, uniformly between the tortillas. Add sliced cilantro to the garnish and pour green sauce.

AIP Cauliflower Pizza with Pesto

Cooking Time: 25 minutes

Serving Size: 1

Calories: 524

Ingredients:

For the Pesto

- ¼ cup olive oil
- 1.5 cups of fresh basil leaves
- 2 cloves of garlic (peeled)
- ½ lemon zest and juice
- Pinch of salt

For the cauliflower pizza base

- Salt to taste
- 2 tablespoon reserved pesto
- ½ teaspoon onion powder
- ½ teaspoon dried oregano
- 1 tablespoon olive oil
- ½ head of cauliflower
- 3 tablespoons of arrowroot flour
- ½ teaspoon garlic powder
- A small quantity of red onion

Method:

1. Using a food processor, create the pesto by mixing the oil, herbs, and garlic with the lime zest of fresh lemon.
2. Season with salt and store it in a pan.
3. Heat the oven to 350°F.

4. Put the trashed cauliflower in a bowl and cook for 6 minutes in the oven, partly sealed, on warm.
5. Remove and tip the cauliflower gently on a clean dish towel or cloth. Allow cooling.
6. Place the cauliflower across the dishcloth and extract as much of the water out as you can.
7. Put the onion powder, arrowroot, dried oregano, garlic powder, olive oil, and salt into a dish.
8. Combine well, so a ball of dough can contain it.
9. Place on a parchment paper-lined tray and mold into a short, thin pizza form. Place it for twenty minutes in the oven.
10. Spread one to two teaspoons of pesto and finish with some finely sliced red onions. Remove from the oven. Instantly serve.

Butternut Squash Noodles with Spinach and Mushrooms

Cooking Time: 15 minutes

Serving Size: 4

Calories: 248

Ingredients:

- 8 ounces of mushrooms
- 1 cup fresh spinach
- Salt and pepper to taste
- 3 tablespoons butter
- 1 medium butternut squash
- 1 tablespoon coconut oil
- 1 shallot (diced)
- 10 fresh sage leaves

Method:

1. Chop off the butternut squash tip, and also the seeds, and set aside for another occasion.

2. Peel the remaining squash until the yellow no longer appears to you.
3. You are expected to have bright orange flesh left.
4. Halve and spiral when you are left with all the noodles.
5. Cook and fry the shallot with coconut oil until it is transparent.
6. Add the mushrooms and fry until the water comes, and the mushrooms start to tan.
7. Combine the spinach and blend until thoroughly heated. To eat, sprinkle with salt and pepper.
8. In the meantime, over a medium-low flame, melt butter in a clear bowl.
9. Add the sage as it starts to boil, and watch closely when cooking.
10. Return the squash noodles to the bowl after a moment, flipping with tongs until the noodles are covered.
11. Add salt and pepper to season and prepare until the noodles are ready.
12. Mix the mushroom and vegetable mixture and eat.

Mushroom Ravioli

Cooking Time: 1 hour 15 minutes

Serving Size: 18

Calories: 240

Ingredients:

Ravioli Dough

- ½ cup tapioca flour
- 1.5 teaspoon sea salt
- 1 cup tiger nut flour
- 1 cup cassava flour
- 2 tablespoon olive oil
- ¾ cup hot water
- 1 cup Tapioca flour
- 2 tablespoon nutritional yeast

- ½ teaspoon ground turmeric

Alternative Dough Recipe:

- 3 tablespoon olive oil
- 2 tablespoon nutritional yeast
- 2 teaspoon of sea salt
- ½ teaspoon ground turmeric
- 3 whole pieces boiled cassava
- 1 cup cassava flour

Mushroom Filling

- 1.5 teaspoon sea salt
- handful fresh parsley
- 2 tablespoon olive oil
- 1.5 tablespoon apple cider vinegar
- 6 cloves garlic
- 2 tablespoon nutritional yeast
- 3 tablespoon coconut cream
- 3 cups mushrooms
- 1 onion

Sauce/Gravy

- 2 tablespoon coconut cream
- ½ teaspoon of sea salt
- 1 tablespoon olive oil
- 2 tablespoon cassava flour
- ¾ cup vegetable stock

Method:

1. Blend Mushrooms with garlic and onions in a food processor. In a medium-hot plate, add the oil and fry until the mushrooms are golden brown.
2. Add yeast, salt, and lemon juice. Cook for 7 minutes.
3. Switch off the heat after adding parsley and coconut cream.

4. Combine all the flour mixture and then blend well with hot water until the dough ball shapes. Make ravioli dough filler.
5. Roll out sheets of dough to 1.6 mm on a gritty surface.
6. Add 1 teaspoon of filling onto pieces of dough evenly spaced throughout.
7. Cover and push gently together with another layer of spaghetti, pushing out the moisture around the filling.
8. Use the ravioli knife or a blade to slice out the ravioli.
9. Cook five minutes in hot, boiled water, just until the ravioli floats to the surface.
10. To make the sauce, heat the oil in the saucepan with the flour to make a cream sauce.
11. Add stock and stir out chunks when the roux has golden brown moderately. Continue whisking over medium-high heat until the mixture has thickened.
12. Add spice and add cream to the end. Serve and eat with fresh parsley garnishing.

AIP No Nightshade Ratatouille from Simple French Paleo

Cooking Time: 55 minutes

Serving Size: 4

Calories: 855

Ingredients:

- 1 tablespoon (minced) fresh rosemary
- 1 teaspoon fine sea salt
- 1 medium yellow summer squash (chopped)
- 1 medium zucchini (chopped)
- ¼ cup olive oil
- 1 large yellow onion (chopped)
- 1 tablespoon dried oregano
- 2 medium golden beets (chopped)
- 3 medium carrots (chopped)
- 4 cloves garlic (minced)

Method:

1. Heat coconut oil over a moderately low flame in a medium skillet.
2. Add beets, vegetables, and cloves.
3. Cover and roast, stirring regularly, for twenty minutes.
4. Combine the cabbage, squash, sweet potato, rosemary, coriander, and sea salt.
5. Continue cooking, uncovered, for about twenty minutes until the vegetables are tender.
6. Season to verify and change the salt per taste. Serve cold or hot.

Vegetable Scramble

Cooking Time: 30 minutes

Serving Size: 3

Calories: 393.8

Ingredients:

- 1 teaspoon of sea salt
- 3 cups red cabbage (chopped)
- ½ cup green onions (chopped)
- 2 tablespoon coconut oil
- 3 cups butternut squash (diced)

Method:

1. Melt the coconut oil over medium-high heat in a frying pan.
2. Attach salt, butternut squash, pepper, and red cabbage.
3. Cover and cook, continually mixing, for fifteen minutes.
4. If required, taste and change the spice.
5. Garnish it with sesame seeds right before serving.

AIP Bok Choy Cauliflower Rice

Cooking Time: 25 minutes

Serving Size: 4

Calories: 858

Ingredients:

- 1 small head of cauliflower
- 2 baby bok choy
- 2 tablespoon coconut oil
- 2 teaspoon of sea salt

Method:

1. Break and slice the cauliflower.
2. Slice the baby Bok Choy finely.
3. Add the olive oil, cauliflower, bok choy, and seasoning to a large frying pan or sauté pan over medium heat.
4. Stir occasionally.
5. For a creamy texture, fry for five minutes, and a smoother texture, fry 10 minutes.

Carrot Raisin Pineapple Salad

Cooking Time: 5 minutes

Serving Size: 4

Calories: 112

Ingredients:

- 1 tablespoon honey
- ¼ cup pineapple
- ¾ cup mayonnaise
- 1 lb. (shredded) carrots
- ½ cup raisins

Method:

1. Add the raisins to a cup of hot water, then rinse and wipe on paper towels.
2. Mix with all the rest of the ingredients. Stir well and eat

Cinnamon Roasted Sweet Potatoes and Cranberries

Cooking Time: 30 minutes

Serving Size: 6

Calories: 156

Ingredients:

- 1 tablespoon coconut oil (melted)
- 1 teaspoon salt
- 1 tablespoon maple syrup
- 2 teaspoons cinnamon
- 6 cups chopped sweet potatoes
- 8-ounce bag of cranberries

Method:

1. Heat the oven to 400 °F.
2. Combine the cranberries, sweet potatoes, coconut oil, and maple syrup in a wide dish.
3. Stir the paste until it reaches the potatoes and berries equally.
4. Then mix ½ teaspoon salt with seasoning and stir to coat uniformly.
5. Place onto a parchment paper-lined baking tray.
6. For 50 minutes, bake until a fork penetrates through the sweet potatoes quickly.
7. Sprinkle with the remaining ¼ tablespoon of oil and remove it from the oven.

Easy Autoimmune Paleo Coleslaw

Cooking Time: 10 minutes

Serving Size: 4

Calories: 214

Ingredients:

- pepper to taste
- 1 head (shredded) cabbage
- 2 tablespoons honey

- fine sea salt
- 1 cup full fat coconut milk
- ¼ cup apple cider vinegar

Method:

1. Mix all ingredients in a bowl and refrigerate for 1 hour.
2. Serve with rice.

Radish Salsa

Cooking Time: 30 minutes

Serving Size: 4

Calories: 12

Ingredients:

- 1 tablespoon squeezed lemon juice
- ground black pepper
- ½ pound radishes
- 2 tablespoons cilantro leaves
- Coarse kosher salt
- 1 clove garlic (crushed)
- 1 jalapeño without ribs and seeds

Method:

1. In the food processor, put the jalapeño, radishes, lemon juice, garlic, and cilantro and process until finely diced.
2. In a shallow cup, move and stir in salt and pepper to fit.
3. Allow twenty minutes to sit in the refrigerator to enable the flavor to develop.

1.2 Poultry and Meat Recipes

Beef Stew with Orange and Cranberries

Cooking Time: 20 minutes

Serving Size: 4

Calories: 481

Ingredients:

- ½ teaspoon salt
- 1 cup cranberries
- 1-kilogram boneless grass-fed beef steak
- 2 cups suitable gelatinous beef broth
- 1 teaspoon cinnamon
- 2 tablespoon Lemon zest
- 1 tablespoon maple syrup
- 1 tablespoon solid fat
- 1 large onion (sliced)
- 1 large bay leaf

Method:

1. Heat oven at 300°F.
2. Cook the beef in batches, slice it on a tray with a serving dish, and put it on one edge.
3. When the meat is golden brown, then cut, apply to the casserole a tablespoon of fat, and then the vegetables.
4. Turn down the heat to the right and steam until visible for 8 minutes or so.
5. If the skillet is just a little too brown and dehydrated at some point, a tablespoon of water can help loosen the moisture, so scrape it off rapidly and add it into the onions before evaporating the moisture.
6. Mix in the cinnamon whenever the onions are soft and fluffy, and simmer for one more moment.

7. Add the golden-brown beef and the rest of the ingredients, except for the cranberries, then combine properly, making sure the liquid covers the meat.
8. Put the lid on, switch the heat up to a boil, and put it in the oven.
9. Heat for 2 hours, or until the meat is entirely crispy.
10. Stir in the cranberries and roast for an extra 15 minutes.

Cornish Hand Pies

Cooking Time: 35 minutes

Serving Size: 8

Calories: 372

Ingredients:

For the Filling:

- 1 tablespoon. oil
- ¼ cup (diced) onion
- ¼ cup (chopped) celery
- 1 garlic clove (crushed)
- ¼ teaspoon (dried) thyme
- ¼ cup (chopped) carrot
- ¼ lb. ground beef

For the Pastry:

- 5 tablespoon shortening
- 5 tablespoon water
- ¼ teaspoon baking soda
- pinch of sea salt
- ¾ cup cassava flour
- ¼ c arrowroot flour

Method:

1. In a pan, melt oil. Add the carrot, onion, and celery. For 2 minutes, fry.

2. Add the thyme and garlic and simmer for an additional 1 minute.
3. Add the beef and fry until it is no longer pink. Stir in a bowl and cool.
4. Preheat the oven to 400 degrees Fahrenheit. Line the parchment paper with a baking tray.
5. Merge the rice, baking soda, and salt in a large dish.
6. Apply the shortening and slice until crispy in the dry ingredients.
7. To shape the batter, add the water and begin to blend. In the pot, knead a couple of times.
8. Break into two balls and roll out each ball between two parchment paper sheets up to ¼ inch longer.
9. Break the dough into pieces with a 3-inch circular pastry cutter and move it to the lined baking sheet with a spoon.
10. On the baking tray, add a tablespoon of stuffing into the center of each round slice.
11. Pull the leftover dough out and cut it in the same manner.
12. Place on the meat base is filling very gently and softly secure the sides with a fork point.
13. Cut a deep hole in the middle of one of the pies carefully with the edge of a sharp blade.
14. Bake for 15 minutes in the preheated oven.

Prosciutto Meatloaf Muffins with Fig Jam

Cooking Time: 40 minutes

Serving Size: 12

Calories: 410

Ingredients:

- 5 oz. AIP-friendly prosciutto
- 2 lbs. ground beef
- 1 tablespoon thyme leaves

- ½ teaspoon granulated garlic
- 2 cups white sweet potato (cubed)
- ½ teaspoon of sea salt

Method:

1. Heat the oven to 350 degrees Fahrenheit.
2. Line twelve muffin cups with pieces of prosciutto that cover the edges and the rim.
3. Place a steamer bucket over a hot water bowl.
4. Put the potatoes, cover, and heat in the basket for 15 minutes till the potatoes are quickly broken apart with a spoon.
5. In a blender, place the cooked sweet potatoes, meat, thyme leaves, and salt.
6. Heat until the potatoes and beef transfer into a paste.
7. Spoon ¼ cup of the meat mixture into each muffin cup lined with prosciutto.
8. Roast for 20 minutes on the middle shelf of the oven.
9. On top of each muffin, spoon 1 teaspoon of Fig Jam and reheat for 2 minutes before the jam starts to caramelize.
10. Remove with additional Fig Jam on the sides and serve wet.

Chicken Taquitos by Predominantly Paleo

Cooking Time: 20 minutes

Serving Size: 4

Calories: 360

Ingredients:

- 1½ cup avocado oil
- 2 cups mashed yucca
- 1 plantain (peeled)
- 1 teaspoon garlic sea salt

For Filling

- 1 onion (diced)

- ¼ teaspoon turmeric powder
- ½ teaspoon garlic powder
- ½ teaspoon onion powder
- 2 organic chicken breasts
- 1 teaspoon of sea salt

For Avocado Dipping Sauce

- Juice of ½ lime
- ¼ cup of coconut milk
- ½ teaspoon garlic sea salt
- 2 avocados
- Large handful (chopped) cilantro

Method:

1. In a tiny skillet, fry the onion with 1 teaspoon of oil until lightly browned, then set aside.
2. In a vigorous blender, take the crushed yucca and mix with the sliced plantain, garlic, salt, and coconut oil until a dough is produced.
3. Take the dough out of the processor and let it cool slightly.
4. Take a small amount of the dough and stretch it to form a tortilla around ¼ thickness between two parchment paper sheets.
5. During the folding phase, making tortillas so dense can cause them to break.
6. Repeat until the baking sheet is full or the entire volume of yucca dough is used.
7. Bake for about fifteen min or until it is easier for the tortillas to deal with.
8. For about twenty minutes or until heated through, reheat chicken breasts in simmering water in a slow cooker while making tortillas.
9. Drain the water from the chicken and move the chicken with the remaining seasonings to a heavy blender.

10. Mix until the chicken is finely sliced and add the onion and sauté.
11. Boost the oven temperature to 425°F.
12. Now bring one prepared tortilla and put the tortilla lengthwise with 1 tablespoon of the flavored chicken and onions combination.
13. Roll the tortilla into a taquito and place it back on the baking sheet lined with parchment. Do the same with the leftover chicken and tortillas.
14. Bake for the next 15 minutes or until it is soft and crispy; to avoid frying, you will need to keep a close eye on them.
15. Place all the dipping sauce components in a food processor or blender with the avocado dipping sauce and eat.

Maple Roasted Chicken and Sweet Potatoes

Cooking Time: 30 minutes

Serving Size: 6

Calories: 430

Ingredients:

- ¼ teaspoon pepper
- fresh thyme for garnish
- 4 chicken breasts
- 8 sprigs fresh thyme
- 2 tablespoon olive oil
- 2 large sweet potatoes
- ¾ teaspoon salt
- 1 yellow onion
- 3 tablespoon maple syrup

Method:

1. Preheat the oven at 400 degrees Fahrenheit.

2. Peel sweet potatoes and slice them into bits about one-inch longer.
3. Chop the onion into around 1-inch bits, approximately.
4. Toss the sweet potatoes, onions, meat, and vegetable oil, in a broad baking dish, a mix of syrup, salt, and pepper.
5. Place the chicken on the sides of the pan, so the liquid cooks and remains moist.
6. Cover with thyme sprigs and put them in the oven on the central rack.
7. Bake, uncovered, for about forty minutes, stirring midway through. (The thyme leaves will start to fall off when they cook)
8. Turn the breast meat side up, top the veggies once the meat is cooked.
9. Reheat for a couple of minutes, till nicely light browned.

Cranberry Pulled Pork

Cooking Time: 25 minutes

Serving Size: 6

Calories: 409

Ingredients:

- 2 tablespoons fresh thyme (chopped)
- 1 cup cranberries
- 1 tablespoon balsamic vinegar
- 2 tablespoon arrowroot flour
- 2 lbs. boneless pork roast
- 1 cup broth
- 2 tablespoon maple syrup
- 1 teaspoon of sea salt
- 2 tablespoon oil
- 1 medium onion (chopped)
- 3 garlic cloves (crushed)
- 1 cup cranberry juice

Method:

1. Sprinkle salt on the meat. Heat oil on high heat in a medium saucepan and fry pork on both sides. Switch to a pressure cooker.
2. Apply the garlic and onions to the pan and fry till the onion is tender, for about five minutes.
3. Mix in thyme, cranberry juice, stock, vinegar, and syrup. In a small saucepan, bring to a gentle boil and then spill over the beef.
4. Add the cranberries in the slow cooker. Heat for 6 minutes on low or 4 on average.
5. Load liquid into a saucepan from a pressure cooker and bring it to a boil.
6. Whisking the arrowroot powder and cold water together will be necessary at this stage. Then add the cranberry solution into it.
7. Continue cooking until the mixture is thick, about 1 minute.
8. Shred the meat in the pressure cooker using two forks.
9. Pour ½ to ¾ of a cup of cranberry paste back into the slow cooker from the small saucepan and blend before serving with the pork belly.
10. Pour the leftover sauce into a serving platter and serve with the pork belly as a side dish.

1.3 Seafood Recipes

Hearty Salmon Chowder

Cooking Time: 45 minutes

Serving Size: 6

Calories: 280

Ingredients:

- 2 small rutabagas

- 1 large bay leaf
- ¾ teaspoon sea salt
- 2 tablespoon solid fat
- 3 sprigs fresh thyme
- ¾ lb. wild salmon fillet
- 2 cups of coconut milk
- 1 small fennel
- 1 large leek
- 1 cup fish bone broth
- chopped curly parsley to garnish
- 2 stalks celery
- 1 small celeriac
- 2 large carrots

Method:

1. In a big pan, heat the fat and insert the thyme and vegetables.
2. Put the lid on top and cook for 25 minutes on a moderate simmer or until soft, mixing once in a while.
3. In the meantime, put the salmon in a wide saucepan with the coconut milk, stock, and bay leaf on medium heat.
4. Bring the fluid to a gentle boil and poach the fish until only tender for 8 minutes.
5. Remove the coconut milkfish, remove the skin and the bay leaf.
6. With the veggies, add the milk into the sauce, bring to a boil and cook for another five minutes or until the rutabaga and vegetables have cooked through.
7. Flake the salmon into large parts, add and heat the vegetables, taking care not to cause the chowder to simmer. To taste, apply sea salt.

5 Minute Broiled Salmon

Cooking Time: 8 minutes

Serving Size: 4

Calories: 208

Ingredients:

- ¼ teaspoon dried oregano
- 2 teaspoon coconut oil
- ¼ teaspoon garlic powder
- ½ teaspoon of sea salt
- ¼ teaspoon black pepper
- Juice from ½ lemon
- 1½ lb. wild salmon filets

Method:

1. Heat the oven and level the baking dish about 5 inches from the heat source.
2. In a cast-iron pan, heat the coconut oil over medium temperature for three minutes until it boils on the broiler pan.
3. When you want crisp salmon skin, this move is essential.
4. Meanwhile, pat the salmon fillets dry.
5. Apply with ½ teaspoon sea salt on the skin line.
6. Turn the fillets over and season the surface with the remaining black pepper, sea salt, oregano, and garlic powder, so they are skin side down.
7. Place the salmon fillets in the pan, until ready.
8. Shift the pan into the oven instantly and broil for five minutes.
9. Remove from the heat before eating and pour the lemon juice over the fillets.

Mini Paleo Salmon Cakes and Lemon Herb Aioli

Cooking Time: 45 minutes

Serving Size: 10

Calories: 74

Ingredients:

- ½ teaspoon ground black pepper
- Lemon wedges
- 2 ¼ cups cooked salmon
- 1 tablespoon lemon juice
- 3 tablespoons capers
- 1 tablespoon Dijon mustard
- 1 teaspoon lemon zest
- ¼ cup mashed sweet potato
- 4 green onions
- 1 tablespoon fresh parsley (chopped)
- 1 egg (beaten)
- ¾ teaspoon sea salt

Lemon Herb Aioli

- 1 tablespoon fresh parsley
- 1 teaspoon fresh dill
- ½ teaspoon Dijon mustard
- ½ cup garlic infused regular olive oil
- 1 egg yolk
- 1 tablespoon fresh lemon juice
- 1 large clove garlic

Method:

1. Heat the oven at 350°F.
2. Add all of the salmon cake components into a big mixing bowl.
3. Use a fork until combined, put everything together.
4. Shape mini patties and put them on the baking tray, around three inches in length.

5. Bake for 25 minutes or until the sides are solid and brown. Be sure that midway through cooking time, turn the patties over in the oven.
6. Create the aioli when the salmon cakes are baking. A blender is the best way to create this, but you can also do this in a mixing bowl, mixer, or hand blender.
7. In a small bowl, put the egg yolk, ½ of the lime juice, and mustard.
8. When the mixture gets thicker, continue whisking it together. Then add the olive oil into it steadily. It is necessary to add oil gradually.
9. Add more oil as the paste thickness increases, until you have a thick, smooth mayo.
10. Along with the parsley, garlic, and dill, add the rest of the lime juice and blend in by hand. If needed, taste and sprinkle with salt.
11. Move the aioli and place it with the salmon cakes in a little dish.
12. For up to a week, put the leftovers in an airtight jar in the refrigerator.

Fig Crusted Salmon

Cooking Time: 30 minutes

Serving Size: 6

Calories: 230

Ingredients:

- ½ tablespoon garlic powder
- ¼ cup of orange juice
- ¼ tablespoon pink Himalayan salt
- ½ cup of water
- ¼ tablespoon cinnamon powder
- 1-pound salmon
- 3 dried figs (chopped)
- 1 date

Method:

1. Heat the oven to 350F
2. Put salmon on baking paper and line on reheating baking paper.
3. Place all other items in a frying pan and bring to a full boil.
4. Make the fig covering. Simmer for five minutes or until much of the liquid is ready for baking.
5. Shift to a food processor for consistent performance.
6. Spread the fig covering thinly on the fish
7. Depending on the salmon parts' size and how much you like your salmon, bake for eighteen minutes.
8. To stop cooking, let the salmon stay on the stove or counters for 4 minutes.
9. Serve with roasted vegetables for a full meal and a raw salad.

Caramelized Salmon

Cooking Time: 30 minutes

Serving Size: 4

Calories: 305

Ingredients:

- 2 Salmon Fillets
- 2 tablespoon Olive oil
- Dash of black pepper
- ¼ cup of coconut sugar
- 1 tablespoon of sea salt

Method:

1. Combine the coconut sugar, salt, and pepper in a little cup.
2. In a medium pan, add coconut oil and heat on medium-high heat.

3. Take the salmon fillets and uniformly add the spice then rub all over.
4. When the pan is heated, put your fillets on each side for about 2 minutes until it is fluffy and thoroughly cooked in the pan.

Baked Parsnip Salmon Cakes

Cooking Time: 20 minutes

Serving Size: 8

Calories: 141.5

Ingredients:

- ½ teaspoon salt
- 2 6 oz. cans of wild salmon
- 2 teaspoon dried dill leaves
- Avocado oil for brushing
- 1 lb. parsnips
- 2 teaspoon garlic powder

Method:

1. Cut and slice off the parsnips and remove the ends.
2. Cut the parsnips, chopping the thick ends in two before slicing via the stems such that all the bits are approximately the same size.
3. Cover with water and bring to a simmer, then boil to turn down the heat.
4. Cook till the parsnips are fork-tender for around 15 to 20 minutes.
5. Wash the parsnips and then let them cool completely before the steam disperses for a couple of minutes.
6. To loosely mix the parsnips around, use a food processor or fork.

7. Remove the salmon and use the crushed parsnips to drip it into the pan. To blend all the items equally, add the dill, garlic, and ginger, then mix.
8. Heat the oven to 425F and use baking paper to line a baking dish.
9. Rub the parchment paper with a little coconut oil.
10. Load the parsnip paste into a ¼ cup to make around 8 equally shaped cakes, then put the rounds on the baking tray, straightening the tops and layering the sides in your palms as appropriate.
11. With a little extra grease, clean the surfaces of the salmon cakes and bake for fifteen minutes.
12. To gently flip the cakes around, use a thin silicone spoon, and return the cakes to the oven until they are slightly browned, for another 10 minutes.
13. With a few lemon wedges, serve immediately

Creamy Cod and Shrimp Chowder

Cooking Time: 45 minutes

Serving Size: 4

Calories: 414

Ingredients:

- 1 lb. cod fillet
- 1 lb. peeled and deveined shrimp
- 1 lb. cauliflower
- 5 cups of seafood stock
- 1 teaspoon dried dill weed
- 1 teaspoon fine sea salt
- 1 13.5 oz. can of coconut milk
- ¾ lb. parsnips
- 1 medium onion, diced
- 4 cloves garlic

Method:

1. Cut the cauliflower into florets finely, then cut the parsnips and slice them.
2. To cut and dispose of the outer membrane, cut the parsnips into pieces and break the cloves of garlic.
3. In a big roasting pan over medium-high heat, add the cauliflower, diced onion, parsnips, garlic, seafood stock, and salt.
4. Carry the stock to boil evenly and continue cooking for about 20 minutes until the veggies are fork-tender.
5. Remove the oven from the heat. Add the coconut milk.
6. To gently thicken the broth until it is creamy and fluffy in texture, use a blender.
7. Mix the dried dill in and transfer the pan to the edge of the stove, bringing it up to a low simmer.
8. Split the bite-sized bits of the cod fillet and transfer them to the sauce, along with the shrimp.
9. Cook for another 2 to 3 minutes until the shrimp is yellow, and the cod is transparent.
10. For a soothing cool edition, serve immediately or cool overnight in the refrigerator!

Prosciutto-Wrapped Cod with Lemon Caper Spinach

Cooking Time: 20 minutes

Serving Size: 2

Calories: 196

Ingredients:

- 2 tablespoon grass-fed butter
- 2 tablespoon capers
- 1 clove garlic
- 4 cups baby spinach
- 14 oz. cod fillets

- 1 teaspoon fresh lemon juice
- Zest of 1 lemon
- Sea salt and pepper
- 1.5 oz. prosciutto

Method:

1. With paper towels, pat fillets dry thoroughly and enable them to move to room temperature.
2. Press them to clean again until they are at room temperature and brush with a little salt and black pepper. Not that much salt now, since it is spicy with prosciutto.
3. Cover the prosciutto fillets.
4. Only cover the strips to make a layer and then tie around the fillets if your prosciutto is in sheets rather than strips.
5. On a level surface, set out the prosciutto, put the fillet on edge, then roll the fillet to seal it.
6. In the oven or another non-stick pan, heat butter over moderate flame.
7. Replace the fillets until the butter is warmed and cook over medium heat on either side or until the salmon flakes can be moved easily with a spoon.
8. Use a lightweight spatula, flip cautiously. Set preparation time depending on the fillets' weight.
9. To a cooling rack, cut the fillets. It inhibits the bottoms from being soggy.
10. Add the garlic to the pot and cook for about thirty seconds, with the burner still on moderate heat.
11. Add capers, spinach, and lemon juice. For around 1-2 minutes, mix and fry only until you have wilted the spinach.
12. Use tongs to transfer the spinach onto dishes. Spray with lemon zest and cover with the cod.

Paleo Fish and Chips

Cooking Time: 10 minutes

Serving Size: 2

Calories: 578

Ingredients:

- 1-pound cod
- avocado oil for frying
- ⅓ cup of water
- pinch of sea salt
- ⅓ cup cassava flour
- ⅓ cup plain kombucha
- ¼ cup tapioca starch

Method:

1. Heat oven to 375 degrees.
2. If a shallow fryer cannot be used, make sure you use a deep pot to prevent splashing and pay particular attention to the heat so that when the fish is inserted, it does not get too warm or drop too far.
3. In a small bowl with a spoon, combine the kombucha, cassava flour, and salt.
4. To form a dense and moist batter, add up to ¼ cup of water.
5. In a different shallow bowl, put the tapioca starch and cover both sides of the cod gently.
6. Put the cod fillets in the batter and begin to cover. Enable it to drain off some of the moisture and then move to the hot oil.
7. Fry for 5 minutes, until it is lightly browned in the batter.
8. Remove from the oil and enable it to soak over a baking tray on a set wire rack.
9. Serve immediately.

Perfect Pan-Fried Scallops and Bacon

Cooking Time: 30 minutes

Serving Size: 2

Calories: 364.2

Ingredients:

- 10 scallops
- pinch of salt
- 1 teaspoon salted butter
- 4 rashers streaky bacon

Method:

1. On medium heat, quickly prepare a frying pan and set out the bacon, hot-fry it so that it begins to turn crispy, and the fat flows into the pan.
2. When the bacon is fried, slightly crispy and golden, lift it out of the pan and place it on a plate on one side.
3. In the bowl, add a tablespoon of butter to the bacon fat and cook softly until the butter begins to soften.
4. Swirl it around the bowl and add the scallops, putting them on a counter like the digits, beginning at 12.
5. When they touch the hot pan, you can see the scallops quickly contract.
6. Allow it to sizzle for about two minutes and then switch each one over in the order you put them.
7. Leave it for the next minute or two to simmer. The bottom should still be moist and golden on the bottom of the scallop.
8. With the creamy-bacon juices and the bacon rashers separately, prepare the scallops. A salad is ideal as it is very light-or served with any summer vegetables such as broccoli or asparagus.

Chapter 2: Snacks, Sweets, and Drink Recipes

2.1 Snack Recipes

Autoimmune Paleo Pumpkin Granola

Cooking Time: 30 minutes

Serving Size: 3 cups

Calories: 270

Ingredients:

- 1 teaspoon nutmeg
- ½ teaspoon of sea salt
- 1½ cup coconut chips
- 1 tablespoon maple syrup
- 2 teaspoon cinnamon
- 1 tablespoon pumpkin puree
- 2 tablespoon coconut oil
- 1 cup chopped raw almonds
- ⅓ cup dried cranberries

Method:

1. Heat the oven to 350F and use parchment paper to cover the baking sheet.
2. In a mixing cup, pour all the dried ingredients and blend.
3. Put in the syrup, coconut oil, pumpkin puree, and mix to coat evenly.
4. Onto the baking dish, spoon the mixture out, and bake for 10 minutes. To ensure that it does not smoke, check the granola.
5. Take it out of the oven and leave to cool. Stock up for a week in the refrigerator and eat on the go over almond cream, paleo pancakes, or as a snack by itself.

Tigernut "Cheese" Crackers

Cooking Time: 25 minutes

Serving Size: 15 to 20

Calories: 35

Ingredients:

- 1 teaspoon of sea salt
- ½ teaspoon black pepper
- ½ teaspoon turmeric powder
- 1 tablespoon gelatin
- 1 tablespoon nutritional yeast
- 1 cup tiger nut flour
- 3 tablespoon coconut oil
- ¼ cup of water

Method:

1. Heat the oven at 350 F. Mix the tiger nut flour, avocado oil, yeast, turmeric, salt, and black pepper in a medium mixing cup. Place aside the combination.
2. Pour ¼ cup of water into a shallow pan of sauces and add it to the pot's top. Spray the gelatin into the water gently and enable 1-2 minutes to develop.
3. To allow the gelatin to melt, switch the heat to medium/low for 2-3 minutes.
4. Remove the pot from the heat quickly and whisk until it foams.
5. To mix, add the gelatin and eggs into the mixture and stir rapidly.
6. Line the parchment paper with a baking dish and put the mixture on the paper.
7. On top of the dough, put another parchment paper sheet and sandwich it between two parchment paper pieces.
8. Compress the dough through the top sheet of parchment paper, using either a rolling pin or your fingertips, until it's thin and straight.

9. Cut the dough into crisps using a pizza cutter. You can even use a chopstick to add holes in the small crackers.
10. Bake the crackers to your taste for 12 minutes or until crispy. Remove from the oven and allow it to cool for removal from the pan before using a spatula.
11. Serve instantly or refrigerate for 1-2 days for a later snack.

Garlic Rosemary Plantain Crackers

Cooking Time: 1 hour 15 minutes

Serving Size: 2 cups

Calories: 220

Ingredients:

- 1 teaspoon granulated garlic
- ½ teaspoon of sea salt
- 2 large, green plantains
- ½ cup of coconut oil
- 2 tablespoon fresh rosemary

Method:

1. Heat the oven to 300°F.
2. Cut a slice from one side of the plantains to another and slice them with the cut.
3. Cut them into big pieces and put them with the olive oil, garlic, rosemary, and salt in a blender.
4. Blend or mix until it forms a slightly dense and crunchy combination.
5. Pour on a baking parchment paper and roll out with either a spatula or some other baking parchment slice and a rolling pin until it is ¼ thick.
6. Bake for ten minutes in the oven. Cut and label with a knife into 1½ crackers.
7. Put them back in the oven and cook for an additional 50 minutes to one hour. When the crisps are medium

brown, and the middle ones are not soft any more, finish frying.

8. You will need to cook these for approximately 20 more minutes to allow them to get fully crispy.

Asian Stuffed Mushrooms

Cooking Time: 15 minutes

Serving Size: 4

Calories: 100

Ingredients:

For the Mushrooms and Stuffing

- 2 tablespoons coconut amino
- 1 teaspoon salt
- 2 green onions
- 2 cloves of garlic
- 20 medium white button mushrooms
- ½ lb. ground chicken
- 1 tablespoon ginger

For the Dipping Sauce

- ½ teaspoon apple cider vinegar
- 4 tablespoons of coconut amino
- 4 cloves of garlic

Method:

1. Merge the chicken, garlic, spring onions, ginger, coconut, and spice in a mixing dish. Mix well.
2. Wash the mushrooms. Pack the meat mixture into the mushrooms with your hands. It may either be cooked or steamed.
3. Combine the garlic, vinegar, amino, and coconut in a shallow bowl to form the dipping sauce.
4. Serve the dipping sauce with the steamed stuffed mushrooms.

Coconut Banana Balls

Cooking Time: 15 minutes

Serving Size: 12

Calories: 79.3

Ingredients:

- 1 banana
- Dash of salt
- Unsweetened cacao powder
- 2 tablespoons coconut oil
- 1 teaspoon vanilla extract
- 2 cups coconut
- 1 tablespoon raw honey

Method:

1. If you want to serve hot, heat the oven to 250F.
2. In a dish, combine all the ingredients properly.
3. Using your hands, shape tiny balls out of the dough.
4. Refrigerate or cook for 20 minutes at 250F.

Spinach Basil Chicken Meatballs Recipe with Plum Balsamic Sauce

Cooking Time: 20 minutes

Serving Size: 24

Calories: 136

Ingredients:

- 3 tablespoons of olive oil
- 1 teaspoon of salt
- 10 basil leaves
- 2 chicken breasts
- ¼ lb. of spinach
- 5 cloves of garlic

Method:

1. Put in a food processor the chicken breasts, salt, spinach, fresh basil, garlic, and coconut oil and blend well.
2. With the meat mixture, produce ping-pong shaped balls.
3. In a deep fryer, heat the oil or the coconut oil and fry the meatballs over medium-high heat for five minutes.
4. Switch and fry for ten minutes more. Ensure they don't melt the meatballs.
5. Meanwhile, put the vinegar, honey, and water in a blender. Blend properly, creating the plum balsamic sauce.
6. For the meatballs, add half the sauce into the deep fryer and turn the fire on.
7. Brown the meatballs-keep turning the meatballs in the mixture until the sauce is ready and cook the meatballs.
8. Check that the meatballs are cooked properly by slicing or using a meat thermometer.
9. With the remaining gravy, prepare the meatballs.

Pan-Fried Apricot Tuna Salad Bites

Cooking Time: 5 minutes

Serving Size: 5

Calories: 140

Ingredients:

- 2 cans of tuna
- 2 tablespoons olive oil
- Sea salt to taste
- 5 apricots
- 1 teaspoon Coconut oil
- 5 blueberries
- 2 tablespoons thyme leaves

Method:

1. Put the olive oil in a saucepan and deep-fry the cut-face down apricot halves, so they are golden brown. Additionally, the apricot halves should be fried directly.
2. Combine the tuna, thyme leaf, coconut oil, and salt in a bowl.
3. Load chunks of the tuna paste on top of the apricot halves using a scoop.
4. Use blueberry on top of each apricot.

AIP Carrot Fries Recipe with Coconut and Cinnamon

Cooking Time: 25 minutes

Serving Size: 2

Calories: 62

Ingredients:

- 1 tablespoon cinnamon powder
- 5 oz. of carrots
- 1 teaspoon ginger powder
- Dash of salt
- 2 tablespoons coconut oil

Method:

1. Preheat the oven to 220C.
2. If your vegetables are frozen, place them in the oven to warm them to room temperature. This avoids the solidification of the coconut oil.
3. Mix the coconut oil, cinnamon, and a sprinkle of salt.
4. Place over a parchment paper-lined with baking sheet.
5. Bake for 20-25 minutes until fries are crispy.
6. Spray on top with more cinnamon and serve.

Baked Pita Chips

Cooking Time: 20 minutes

Serving Size: 2

Calories: 130

Ingredients:

- 3 tablespoons olive oil
- ¼ cup arrowroot
- 4 tablespoons cold water
- ¼ cup tapioca or cassava flour

Method:

1. Preheat the oven to 200C.
2. Using your palms, combine all the items properly.
3. Put and roll flat on a sheet of parchment paper.
4. To shape tiny 1-inch circles, mark the dough.
5. Place in the oven and bake for 15 minutes.
6. Cool and serve.

Paleo Popcorn Meatballs

Cooking Time: 25 minutes

Serving Size: 2

Calories: 52

Ingredients:

- 1 lb. Grass-fed ground beef
- 6 tablespoon hot water
- 1 cup of solid cooking fat
- 6 tablespoon grass-fed gelatin
- 3 tablespoon cold water
- ½ teaspoon of sea salt
- ½ teaspoon ground turmeric
- ½ teaspoon garlic powder
- ½ teaspoon garlic powder
- 1 cup tapioca flour
- ½ teaspoon of sea salt

Method:

1. Heat the cooking fat over medium-high heat in a mini frying pan.

2. Combine the ground beef with ¼ tablespoon of salt and ½ teaspoon of the garlic powder in a mixing dish.
3. When mixed with ground beef, make an average meatball.
4. Take another mixing bowl to blend the tapioca flour, salt, garlic powder, then turmeric until all of the meat has been formed into balls.
5. Then, put the gelatin in a small bowl and coat it with cold water.
6. Leave it for about a moment to settle down.
7. Then pour the hot water over the gelatin surface and stir till the gelatin is thoroughly mixed and wet.
8. Transform the heating fat to medium-high temperatures.
9. Take the balls and add them in the mixture of flour, then drop them in the gelatin combination and dredge them again in the flour mix before dipping them into the cooking oil.
10. Use a rubber spatula to move them around and ensure that they are already cooked.
11. Lift them with a spatula from the frying pan after 5 minutes and put them on a metal cooling rack.
12. When all the meatballs are ready, repeat this. Serve and eat with your choice of dipping sauce.

No-Bake Blueberry Pie Energy Bites

Cooking Time: 15 minutes

Serving Size: 5

Calories: 34

Ingredients:

- ½ cup coconut butter
- 1 tablespoon coconut oil
- 1 ¼ cup blueberries
- ½ cup coconut flakes

- Sea salt
- 1 tablespoon honey (optional)
- 1 teaspoon lemon juice
- ½ teaspoon cinnamon

Method:

1. Simmer the berries, coconut sugar, and lemon juice for ten minutes in a frying pan over medium-low heat, mixing every few minutes so that the sugar does not burn.
2. Add the cinnamon and ¼ teaspoon of salt. In a pan, set aside.
3. Rinse out the casserole.
4. In the frying pan, heat the coconut butter over medium heat. Add coconut oil, coconut tiny pieces, and a touch of sea salt to taste.
5. Pour a combination of coconut butter into a silicone muffin mold. Freeze when firm, for twenty minutes.
6. Pour the blueberries uniformly over the surface of the coconut.
7. Refrigerate for two hours or overnight.
8. Place additional cinnamon, powdered coconut milk, or lemon zest on it.

Sweet and Savory Fried Plantains

Cooking Time: 30 minutes

Serving Size: 3

Calories: 102

Ingredients:

For the Sweet Plantains:

- ¼ teaspoon cinnamon
- 1 tablespoon Artisanal Coconut Butter
- 1 tablespoon coconut oil
- 1 yellow plantain

For the Savory Plantains:

- ¼ teaspoon garlic powder
- sea salt to taste
- 1 yellow plantain
- 1 tablespoon Epic Duck Fat

Method:

1. Slice the plantains and peel them.
2. Heat duck fat in one pan and avocado oil in the other skillet over medium heat.
3. Pan-fry pieces of plantain for 2 minutes on either side, taking care not to smoke.
4. Remove from the fire to cool to room temperature on a paper towel-lined pan, then shift each batch to a cup.
5. Add cinnamon and mix with molten coconut butter in a cup. Sprinkle with garlic powder and salt on the other side. Cover and stir.
6. Serve hot and eat immediately.

Cauliflower Dip

Cooking Time: 30 minutes

Serving Size: 2

Calories: 52.4

Ingredients:

- Sea salt, to taste
- Radishes and cucumber sticks
- 3 cloves of garlic (unpeeled)
- ½ head of cauliflower
- 3 tablespoons of olive oil
- 2 tablespoons of lemon juice

Method:

1. Preheat the oven to 200 degrees Celsius.

2. In a cup, put the cauliflower florets and mix in two tablespoons of olive oil.
3. On a greased baking dish, lay them flat.
4. Take the garlic cloves as they are and lock them inside a small foil packet in which no air can enter.
5. To allow roasting, roast in the oven for 30 minutes, tossing the cauliflower after fifteen minutes.
6. Take the fried, caramelized cauliflower florets and bring them into a mini mixing bowl.
7. Open the garlic foil package cautiously and push into the same processor.
8. Add lemon juice and the extra tablespoon of olive oil and combine the mixture into a creamy puree. Season salt to the taste.
9. Serve fresh, with cleaned cucumber and radish sticks with the roasted cauliflower sauce, or any other veggies that you would prefer.

Beetroot Dip

Cooking Time: 15 minutes

Serving Size: 2

Calories: 37

Ingredients:

- 1 teaspoon lemon juice
- Pinch of salt
- 2 tablespoons of fresh cilantro
- 3 beets

Method:

1. Boil the beets until they are tender and then slice. If the beets are already baked, then this stage can be skipped.
2. In a mixer, put all the ingredients and combine well.

2.2 Sweets and Dessert Recipes

AIP Chocolate Chip Cookies (Coconut Free)

Cooking Time: 40 minutes

Serving Size: 12

Calories: 153

Ingredients:

- ½ teaspoon Salt
- ¼ cup Chocolate Chips
- 1 teaspoon Baking Soda
- ½ teaspoon Cream of Tartar
- ¾ cup Arrowroot Starch
- ¼ cup Cassava Flour
- 2 tablespoons Maple Syrup
- ¼ cup Maple Sugar
- ½ cup Palm Shortening
- ¾ teaspoon Vanilla Powder
- 2 tablespoons Gelatin

Method:

1. Preheat oven to 350 degrees.
2. Rub over a large baking sheet with one tablespoon of palm shortening.
3. Blend the wet ingredients in a large mixing bowl, and use a hand-held mixer to produce and shorten the maple syrup.
4. In a small mixing cup, add all the dry ingredients and whisk to coat.
5. Pour the dry ingredients into wet ingredients and mix. Then bring in the chocolate chips using the hand mixer to blend.

6. Create twelve dough balls and place them on the baking sheet.
7. Put it on for 12 minutes in the oven. Remove from the oven and then cool before eating, for another 20 minutes.

AIP Chocolate Banana Cookies with Glaze

Cooking Time: 35 minutes

Serving Size: 8

Calories: 181

Ingredients:

- 3 bananas
- ½ teaspoon baking soda
- ½ cup carob powder
- ¼ cup tiger nut flour
- ¼ teaspoon of sea salt
- ½ cup coconut butter
- ¼ cup of water

Optional Glaze

- 1 tablespoon maple syrup
- 2 pinches sea salt
- ¼ cup coconut oil melted
- 2 tablespoons carob powder roasted

Method:

1. Preheat the oven to 350 degrees Celsius. Grease a large sheet of cookies, or cover them with parchment paper.
2. Combine the dry ingredients in a wide bowl: carob powder, tiger nut powder, baking powder, and sea salt.
3. Mix the banana, peanut butter, and warm water in the blender.
4. Push the button for 15 seconds at the lowest speed and boost to medium-low speed for another 15 seconds, scratching the sides once.
5. Add wet ingredients into dry ingredients. At medium speed, mix with the portable mixer.
6. Use the large cookie scoop on the prepared cookie sheet to portion the cookie batter.
7. To flatten each cookie slightly, wet three fingers: Dip three fingers into warm water. Push the mounded (cookie dough) to dip the fingers back into the water and smooth the surfaces.
8. Bake for about 20 minutes in a preheated oven. Remove and cool fully from the oven.
9. If you intend to glaze them, ice the cookies in the refrigerator or fridge.

Bacon Chocolate Chip Deep Dish Skillet Cookie

Cooking Time: 25 minutes

Serving Size: 8

Calories:

Ingredients:

- ½ cup palm shortening
- 1 tablespoon grass-fed gelatin
- 1 teaspoon baking soda
- 3 tablespoon pure maple syrup
- 3 tablespoon coconut sugar
- ½ cup chocolate chunks
- ¼ cup arrowroot starch
- ¼ cup coconut flour
- 1 teaspoon pure vanilla
- 4 slices cooked bacon (chopped)
- ½ teaspoon cream of tartar
- ½ teaspoon of sea salt

Method:

1. Preheat the oven to 350F.
2. Add shortening, honey, sugar, and vanilla in a big dish. Place aside.
3. Stir flour, gelatin, baking powder, tartar cream, and salt in a medium-scale bowl until mixed. Add flour mixture to wet slowly and blend well to combine.
4. Stir in bits of bacon and chocolate.
5. Insert into an 8-inch cast-iron pan that is greased with shortening and spray with sea salt. Bake for 14 minutes for a rubbery base.
6. Bake for 17 minutes for a cookie that is entirely cooked through that can be sliced into squares.
7. Remove from the oven and let it cool slowly before serving.
8. Do not attempt to cut the cookies before they are cold.

AIP Ginger Cookies

Cooking Time: 40 minutes

Serving Size: 12

Calories: 163.23

Ingredients:

- ¾ cup palm shortening
- 1 teaspoon ground cinnamon
- 2 teaspoons ground ginger
- ¼ cup maple sugar
- ¾ cup arrowroot starch
- ¼ cup cassava flour
- 2 tablespoon gelatins
- 1 teaspoon baking soda
- ½ teaspoon cream of tartar
- ¾ teaspoon vanilla powder
- ½ teaspoon salt

Method:

1. To 350 degrees, heat the oven. Rub over a large baking sheet with one tablespoon of palm shortening.
2. Use a handheld blender, mix the shortening, and molasses to incorporate the wet ingredients into a large mixing cup.
3. Combine all the dry ingredients in a small mixing bowl and swirl to combine, then add the wet ingredients into the big mixing bowl. Stir to blend.
4. Create 12 dough balls and place them on the baking sheet.
5. Push down softly on each ball, using the bottom of a bottle.
6. For 10 minutes, put the baking sheet in the oven.
7. Remove from the oven and then cool before using for another 10 minutes.

Christmas Cut Out Sugar Cookies

Cooking Time: 30 minutes

Serving Size: 7

Calories:

Ingredients:

For the cookies

- ¼ cup maple syrup
- ½ teaspoon baking soda
- 1 tablespoon vital proteins gelatin
- ½ teaspoon vanilla extract
- ¾ cup tapioca starch
- ½ cup tiger nut flour
- ¼ cup palm shortening

For the green frosting

- 2 tablespoon light-colored honey
- ½ teaspoon Matcha powder
- 1 tablespoon arrowroot starch
- ¼ cup palm shortening

For the yellow frosting

- 1 tablespoon light-colored honey
- ¼ teaspoon turmeric powder
- 2 teaspoon arrowroot starch
- 2–3 tablespoon palm shortening

Method:

1. Heat oven to 350 degrees Fahrenheit and use parchment paper to cover a baking sheet especially greased with coconut oil or other items. Just put aside.
2. Combine the dried components in a large mixing dish.
3. Fill the palm shortening and maple syrup together in a different bowl. Add the mixture to the flour mixture.
4. Stir in the vanilla extract until a dough is formed, and the ingredients are mixed.
5. On a parchment paper, move the dough. Take about half of dough at a time and compress to about ¼ inch thick.

6. To cut the dough into the perfect form, use a cookie cutter and pull the fingers around the cookie cutter away from the excess dough.
7. On the baking sheet, move the shaped cookie dough. With the remaining of the dough, repeat the process. There are around 6-7 cookies you can have.
8. Spread the cookies uniformly on the baking sheet and bake for 15 minutes in the oven or until the cookies are lightly nicely browned.

AIP Snickerdoodles

Cooking Time: 20 minutes

Serving Size: 6

Calories: 296

Ingredients:

- ¼ cup collagen
- ½ teaspoon cinnamon
- ¼ teaspoon of sea salt
- 1 teaspoon vanilla extract
- 1 teaspoon apple cider vinegar
- 1 cup tiger nut flour.
- ¼ cup honey
- ½ teaspoon baking soda
- ¼ cup arrowroot flour
- ½ cup of coconut oil

Method:

1. Heat oven to 350 degrees Fahrenheit.
2. Line a big sheet of cookies with parchment paper.
3. Stir together the dried ingredients in a medium-sized bowl: tiger nut flour, arrowroot, collagen, baking powder, cinnamon, and salt.
4. Add wet ingredients. To blend, use a portable mixer, without over-mixing.

5. To split dough on a lined baking sheet, use the baking scoop.
6. Bake until the sides are light brown and the tops are softly tinged for 8 minutes. Enable slightly to cool before eating.

Paleo Pumpkin Snickerdoodles

Cooking Time: 20 minutes

Serving Size: 7

Calories:

Ingredients:

- 2 teaspoon cinnamon (divided)
- 1 ½ tablespoon coconut sugar
- 3 tablespoon pumpkin puree
- ¾ cup tiger nut flour
- ¼ teaspoon baking soda
- ¼ cup maple syrup
- ½ cup arrowroot starch
- 1 tablespoon gelatin
- ¼ cup of coconut oil

Method:

1. Heat the oven to 375 F and use thinly greased parchment paper to cover a baking sheet.
2. Combine the tiger nut flour, starch, gelatin, and baking powder until well mixed.
3. Stir in the olive oil, syrup, pumpkin pie spice, and 1 teaspoon of cinnamon. To mix before a dough forms, stir well.
4. Combine 1 teaspoon of cinnamon along with the coconut sugar in a small bowl or tray. Put aside.
5. Roll the dough into tiny 7 balls. In the cinnamon-sugar mixture, roll every ball until lightly coated.

6. Put the dough balls to the baking sheet and press gently on the cookies with your palm, making sure the cookies are equally spread.
7. In the preheated oven, bake the cookies for 10 minutes or until thoroughly baked.
8. Remove from the oven and allow to cool slowly.
9. Immediately eat or place in an airtight jar for 2 days in the refrigerator.

Strawberry Pie

Cooking Time: 20 minutes

Serving Size: 8

Calories: 291

Ingredients:

- 3 tablespoons Arrowroot Starch
- Mint leaves, garnish
- 1 Pie Crust, 9 inches
- ¾ cups Water
- 1 cup Honey
- ¾ cups Apple Juice
- 3 cups Fresh Strawberries
- 3 tablespoons Gelatin

Method:

1. With a fork, poke the bottom layer of the piecrust and bake according to the instructions.
2. And let it cool. Set aside 1 cup of strawberries and purée.
3. In the pie crust, put the remainder of the strawberries.
4. Over the water, spray the gelatin.
5. Stir to blend and set aside.
6. In a shallow saucepan, add the pureed strawberries, juices, honey, and salt, then mix to blend.

7. Heat until cooked over medium-high heat, reduce the heat a little and boil for around five minutes, until thickened.
8. Remove from the fire and spray in the saucepan with the arrowroot starch and gelatin combination and shake.
9. Pour a combination of strawberry gelatin over the strawberries.
10. Refrigerate for a minimum of 4 hours, or until the pie is set.
11. Serve with healthy mint leaves and extra strawberries.

Healthy Caramelized Apples

Cooking Time: 20 minutes

Serving Size: 4

Calories: 211

Ingredients:

- ½ tablespoon ground cinnamon
- ½ teaspoon salt
- Shredded coconut
- 4 apples peeled
- 4 tablespoons maple syrup
- 2 tablespoons coconut oil

Method:

1. Melt oil on the medium temperature in a large skillet.
2. To the pan, add the apples.
3. While stirring frequently, let them sauté in the pan until lightly browned, about five minutes total. Try to stir for sometimes.
4. Stir in the syrup, salt, and cinnamon, then decrease the heat to moderate.
5. Let it boil for about five minutes until the apples are tender. Stir time to time.
6. If needed, eat warm with shredded coconut.

AIP Pumpkin Pudding

Cooking Time: 20 minutes

Serving Size: 6

Calories: 95

Ingredients:

- ¼ teaspoon ground cinnamon
- ¼ teaspoon ground ginger
- 1 15 ounces can pumpkin puree
- ¼ teaspoon ground cloves
- Dash of sea salt
- ½ teaspoon vanilla powder
- 1 15 ounces can coconut milk
- 1 tablespoon gelatin powder
- ½ cup honey

Method:

1. In a medium mixing cup, apply the gelatin to the coconut milk and stir until mixed. Set aside to let grow for approximately 15 minutes.
2. In a large frying pan, add the remaining ingredients.
3. Let cook over medium heat until the pumpkin paste is cooked through, and the pan's edges begin to bubble. Remove from the flame.
4. Next, add a combination of coconut milk. Stir to make sure it's thoroughly mixed, and there are no gelatin chunks.
5. Load the pudding solution into a bowl and cover well and let it stay for around 3 hours in the fridge to settle.

Paleo Vegan Chocolate Mousse

Cooking Time: 13 minutes

Serving Size: 4

Calories:

Ingredients:

- 3 tablespoons coconut oil
- 1 14-ounce can full-fat coconut milk
- 1 teaspoon vanilla extract
- 1 ½ to 2 tablespoons of cocoa powder
- ¼ teaspoon salt
- 100 grams pitted dates

Method:

1. Scoop out from the can of coconut milk except for ¼ cup of coconut water and put the ingredients in a small container.
2. In a smoothie, use the remaining 1/3 cup of coconut water.
3. Heat it in such a way that it's molten and not stiff anymore.
4. In a high-powered blender, place that and the rest of the ingredients. Blend for around 1 minute and, to taste, add extra cocoa.
5. Pour into desserts cups until thoroughly mixed, and no pieces of dates remain visible.
6. To strengthen up, rest for at least 2 hours. For up to two days, refrigerate leftovers.

AIP Chocolate Marshmallows

Cooking Time: 30 minutes

Serving Size: 24

Calories: 48

Ingredients:

- ¼ teaspoon Salt
- ½ teaspoon Vanilla Powder
- 1 cup Honey
- 4 tablespoons Gelatin
- 2 tablespoons Carob Powder

Method:

1. With the whip extension, prepare the standing mixer.
2. To combine, add the half cup of water into the mixing bowl, apply the gelatin, and then whisk slowly. Set aside.
3. In a shallow saucepan, add in another half cup of water, salt, and honey.
4. Get the water and honey mixture to a boil gradually.
5. Then let it simmer while stirring for around 10 min at a full boil.
6. With the gelatin solution, gently add the honey blend into the bowl.
7. Switch the mixer on to moderate as the mixture of honey is poured.
8. Switch the mixer on maximum for another 10 minutes until the honey paste is added, or until the texture of the marshmallow cream forms a heavy cream.
9. For the last couple of minutes of whipping, add the vanilla and carob.
10. Cover a 9×13-inch baking sheet with parchment paper, leaving enough on the edges to be able to pick up.
11. Pour into the lined tray as the marshmallows are whipped.
12. Smooth the surface with a spatula, so it is even.
13. Let them stay for Eight hours or overnight at ambient temperature.
14. Remove the marshmallows softly from the pan by either tossing the pan onto a cutting board or raising it out with the parchment.
15. Break the marshmallows into bits with a sharp knife, cookie-cutter, or blade.
16. If you need to stack the marshmallows, store them in an airtight jar using parchment paper.

2.3 Drinks Recipes

Avocado Green Smoothie

Cooking Time: 5 minutes

Serving Size: 1

Calories: 189.7

Ingredients:

- 1 handful of greens
- 1 cup ice
- ½ cup of coconut milk
- ½ ripe avocado
- 1 ripe banana

Method:

1. In the blender, put the avocado, ice, and banana.
2. Cover with the greens of preference.
3. Blend until creamy (if you are having trouble mixing it, add extra almond milk or water).

Blueberry Kale Smoothie

Cooking Time: 4 minutes

Serving Size: 1

Calories: 297

Ingredients:

- 1 cup of baby kale
- 1 tablespoon gelatin
- 1 large ripe banana
- 1 cup of milk of choice
- ½ cup of frozen blueberries

Method:

1. Put in your mixer with all the items and whiz up until absolutely smooth.

Blueberry Coconut Yogurt Smoothie

Cooking Time: 5 minutes

Serving Size: 2

Calories: 161

Ingredients:

- ½ teaspoon vanilla extract
- Stevia to taste
- 10 blueberries
- 1 pot of coconut yogurt
- 1 cup of coconut milk

Method:

1. In the blender, combine all the ingredients and mix very well.
2. Enjoy a simple and healthy snack or brunch.

Cranberry Smoothie

Cooking Time: 4 minutes

Serving Size: 1

Calories: 140.2

Ingredients:

- ½ cup of cranberry sauce
- 1 medium ripe banana
- 1 cup of coconut milk

Method:

1. In a mixer, put all of the ingredients and combine them for two minutes.
2. Serve with breakfast.

Orange Cinnamon Ginger Tea

Cooking Time: 2 minutes

Serving Size: 1

Calories: 11

Ingredients:

- 1 slice of ginger
- 2 cups boiling water
- 1 cinnamon stick
- 2 slices of orange

Method:

1. Mix all the ingredients in a big mug and add hot boiling water into it.
2. For five minutes, ferment and enjoy.

AIP Coffee

Cooking Time: 5 minutes

Serving Size: 1

Calories: 33

Ingredients:

- 1 tablespoon chicory powder
- 1 date
- 3 cups of water
- 1 tablespoon dandelion root
- 1 tablespoon carob powder

Method:

1. In a shallow saucepan, mix all the ingredients and bring them to a boil.
2. Lower the heat and give five minutes for the mixture to boil.
3. Withdraw from flame, strain, and drink.

Turmeric Ginger Lime Tea

Cooking Time: 5 minutes

Serving Size: 1

Calories: 13.2

Ingredients:

- 1 small turmeric root
- 1 piece of ginger
- 1 lime, sliced into large slices

Method:

1. Place 1 lemon slice in a big tea kettle, along with all the turmeric and ginger bits.
2. Pour the boiling water in the tea kettle.
3. For five minutes, let the tea brew.
4. Then let it cool again and chill the tea for an iced flavor.

Lemon, Ginger, Honey Tea

Cooking Time: 5 minutes

Serving Size: 1

Calories: 51.0

Ingredients:

- 3 thin slices of ginger
- ½ lemon cut 3 slices
- Honey to taste
- 1 cup boiling water

Method:

1. Put all ingredients into the cup.
2. Dry only for five minutes. Mix and Serve.

Watermelon Agua Fresca with Mint, Ginger, and Lime

Cooking Time: 10 minutes

Serving Size: 9

Calories: 69

Ingredients:

- 3-inch piece of fresh ginger
- 8 sprigs of fresh mint
- Juice of 6 limes
- 9 cups seedless watermelon chunks

To serve:

- Lime slices
- Fresh mint
- Sparkling water
- Coarse sea salt

Method:

1. Fill the processor about ¾ full of watermelon pieces under the peak fill line, then add the lemon, ginger, and fresh mint.
2. Mix until there is watermelon juice with no parts remaining.
3. Over a large bowl, put a fine-mesh sieve and pour the watermelon juice through to strain out the liquid on one at the moment.
4. To stir up and press down each time on the pulp, use a fork, then extract and discard it.
5. Repeat until you have strained all of the juice.
6. To the mixer, add the rest of the watermelon, and squeeze it. If all of the watermelons are juiced and pulp clear, repeat the mixing and squeezing process.
7. Refrigerate the watermelon juice for at least three hours until it is well chilled.

Raspberry Lime Ice

Cooking Time: 5 minutes

Serving Size: 2

Calories: 100

Ingredients:

- A few frozen raspberries to top the drinks
- 35 oz. Coconut Water
- 1 medium lime
- 1 tablespoon honey
- 2 cups of Raspberries
- ¼ teaspoon ground cinnamon power

Method:

1. Place 1 cup of coconut water aside and chill the remainder in the ice cube trays.
2. In a medium saucepan, add the coconut water, berries, half of the lemon juice, and cinnamon and bring to a boil.
3. For three minutes, let it simmer and taste the sauce.
4. If needed, add the honey and put it in a container and set it to chill in the refrigerator.
5. Drop the ice cubes of coconut water (they will be messy) and put them in a blender to smash them into a slushy drink.
6. Fill a cup with the crushed ice and then pour the raspberry syrup on top. Cover with raspberries and pieces of frozen lemon.

Cucumber Lime Water

Cooking Time: 5 minutes

Serving Size: 1

Calories: 10

Ingredients:

- 1.5 liters of water
- 1 cucumber
- 1 lime

Method:

1. Chop and then carve the cucumber into ¼ inch thick strips.
2. Add to the jug and Squeeze 1 lemon into the juice.
3. Add the water and combine.
4. Let it rest overnight in your freezer.

Refreshing Coconut Water Green Drink

Cooking Time: 5 minutes

Serving Size: 2

Calories: 18

Ingredients:

- 1 small cucumber, (washed, sliced, and chopped)
- 10 drops liquid stevia
- ice
- 2 cups of coconut water
- 1 teaspoon (grated) ginger
- ½ cup fresh lemon juice
- 1 large bunch parsley (chopped)

Method:

1. There are several ways you can make this. It tastes tasty either way you make it.
2. Dice cucumber and the parsley and add to a pot. Add the stevia, lime juice, coconut water, and ice.
3. Mix thoroughly with a tight-fitting lid, until mixed. Instantly serve.
4. You will get a somewhat new salad at the bottom of the bowl when you're finished with the cocktail.
5. Add all the ingredients, except for the ice, into a processor and pulse to mix.
6. Pour ice over and drink. If you want it to feel more of a slushy form, add the perfect consistency to some ice and mix.

Cucumber Basil Ice Cubes

Cooking Time: 15 minutes

Serving Size: 2

Calories: 34

Ingredients:

- Juice from ¼ lime
- 5 small basil leaves
- ¼ cup of water
- 1 cucumber (peeled and cut into large chunks)

Method:

1. Place all ingredients in the mixer and mix it properly.
2. Strain the puree and pipe into large ice cube trays or molds with the resulting juice.
3. To make this meal, save the remaining cucumber particles.
4. For 5 hours, ice the trays until firm.
5. Use the ice cubes to make cocktails, apply them to sparkling water to taste the beverage or vodka for a frozen vodka cocktail filled with simple cucumber basil.

Berry Fizz Mocktail

Cooking Time: 5 minutes

Serving Size: 1

Calories: 212

Ingredients:

- 3 oz. tart cherry juice
- 8 raspberries
- 2.5 oz. pomegranate juice
- Sparkling water
- A squeeze of fresh lime juice

Method:

1. Gently press the raspberries into the lemon juice, apply the raspberries and lemon juice to a small pint-sized container, and use a cocktail muddler.
2. Apply the juices of the tart cherry and pomegranate to the container.
3. Shake to mix and freeze the juices and place the lid on the container to add a few ice cubes.
4. Then remove the lid and finish off the drink with fizzy water.
5. Garnish with raspberries and a lemon slice.

Strawberry, Honey, and Lime Spritzer

Cooking Time: 10 minutes

Serving Size: 2

Calories: 15

Ingredients:

Strawberry Honey and Lime Puree

- ¼ cup of raw honey
- Zest from 1 lime
- 1 lb. of ripe strawberries (washed and chopped)

Strawberry Honey and Lime Spritzer

- Ice
- Lime wedge to garnish
- 1.5 ounces of vodka
- Sparkling water
- ¼ cup Strawberry Honey and Lime Puree
- Juice from ½ a lime

Method:

1. Wash strawberries and chop. Set aside in a heatproof dish.
2. Quantify your raw honey out and apply it with your lemon zest to a shallow saucepan.

3. Warm the honey till the mixture begins to bubble over low flame.
4. Allow it to bubble when stirring for 2 minutes and then extract it from the flame.
5. Over the strawberries, add the warm honey and lemon syrup and whisk together until all your strawberries are coated.
6. Enable a minimum of 20 minutes for this combination to sit.
7. The liquid will continue to consume your strawberries and become warm and syrupy.
8. You need to add them to a processor until the strawberries are done.
9. Mix until it turns into a puree. This would only take about 2 minutes.
10. You will need a bottle of ice, half the lemon, and a shot of vodka to complete your drink. The sparkling water would be essential to you.
11. Pour the puree over the ice cubes into the bottom of the container.
12. Now put your liquor shot. You should add ½ cup of lime juice if you want your drink to be slightly on the sour side.
13. Of sparkling mineral water, fill the remainder of your glass and mix.
14. If you are going to make these non-alcoholics, skip the vodka, then repeat all the other procedures.
15. Garnish with a healthy wedge of lime and enjoy the drink.

Creamy Orange Julius

Cooking Time: 10 minutes

Serving Size: 1

Calories: 100

Ingredients:

- 2 tablespoon honey
- Ice cubes
- 4 medium-sized oranges
- 1 tablespoon vanilla
- 1 can of coconut milk

Method:

1. Peel the oranges and de-seed them.
2. Add all of the liquid ingredients to a processor and mix until creamy.
3. Then, add and mix as many ice cubes for the optimal consistency. Serve cold.

2.4 Recipes for Sauces, Condiments, Staples, and Bases

Spicy Guacamole Sauce

Cooking Time: 10 minutes

Serving Size: 2

Calories: 175

Ingredients:

- ½ jalapeño
- ¼ teaspoon of sea salt
- ¼ medium white onion (chopped)
- ¼ cup cilantro (packed)
- ½ avocado
- 1 small garlic clove (chopped)
- Juice from ½ lime

Method:

1. In your mixer or food processor, mix the items.
2. Blend for 2 minutes until smooth.

Cauliflower Nacho Cheese Sauce

Cooking Time: 10 minutes

Serving Size: 2

Calories: 187

Ingredients:

- ¼ cup raw cashews
- ½ cup of water
- 3 tablespoons nutritional yeast
- ½ medium cauliflower (minced)
- 2 tablespoons hot sauce
- ¼ teaspoon salt

Method:

1. At 375 degrees, bake the cauliflower for twenty minutes.
2. Add to your processor the roasted cauliflower and all the ingredients and blend until full and creamy.

Jalapeno Cilantro Chimichurri

Cooking Time: 5 minutes

Serving Size: 2

Calories: 140

Ingredients:

- ½ jalapeno (deseeded)
- ¼ cup red wine vinegar
- 1 large garlic clove (minced)
- 1 teaspoon oregano
- ½ teaspoon of sea salt
- 1 ½ cups cilantro
- ½ cup olive oil

Method:

1. In your mixer or food processor, mix the items.
2. Blend for 2 minutes until smooth.

Cashew Coconut Curry

Cooking Time: 10 minutes

Serving Size: 3

Calories: 297

Ingredients:

- 1 ½ tablespoon red curry paste
- ½ cup of coconut milk
- 1 small garlic clove
- ½ tablespoon cocoa amino
- ½ cup raw cashews
- Juice from ½ lime
- ¼ teaspoon salt

Method:

1. In your mixer or food processor, mix the items.
2. Blend for 2 minutes until smooth.

Honey-less Mustard Sauce

Cooking Time: 15 minutes

Serving Size: 2

Calories: 44

Ingredients:

- ¼ teaspoon salt
- ¼ cup avocado oil
- 1 cup pitted dates, (soaked)
- ¼ cup Dijon mustard
- ¼ cup of water

Method:

1. In a bowl, put the dates and fill them with hot water.
2. For ten minutes, let them soak.

3. Pour the water from the dates and apply them to your processor and all the rest of the ingredients and blend until smooth.

Creamy Bacon Mushroom

Cooking Time: 25 minutes

Serving Size: 2

Calories: 223

Ingredients:

- 1 small shallot
- ½ cup chicken stock
- ¼ teaspoon salt and pepper
- 1 teaspoon fresh thyme
- ¼ cup raw cashews
- 6 cremini mushrooms
- 2 slices of bacon

Method:

1. In a medium-sized grill, cook the bacon and mushroom together over medium-high heat till the mushrooms are golden brown, and the bacon is crunchy for about ten minutes.
2. Add the shallot, then cook for about two minutes.
3. To your mixer, switch the bacon and mushrooms and add the remaining items.
4. Blend until plump and smooth.

Almond Lime Satay

Cooking Time: 10 minutes

Serving Size: 3

Calories: 110

Ingredients:

- Juice from 1 lime

- ¼ teaspoon salt
- ½ cup of coconut milk
- 1 tablespoon cocoa amino
- 6 tablespoons roasted almond butter
- 1 small garlic clove

Method:

1. In a medium-sized cup, mix the items.
2. Combine with a hand mixer.

Carrot Ketchup

Cooking Time: 20 minutes

Serving Size: 2

Calories: 196

Ingredients:

- ¼ teaspoon garlic powder
- ¼ teaspoon ground ginger
- 12 ounces carrot
- 2 tablespoons apple cider vinegar
- ½ teaspoon onion powder
- ½ teaspoon of sea salt
- 6 ounces beet (chopped)
- ¼ cup apple juice
- 3 tablespoons honey

Method:

1. On the base of a wide stockpot, put a steamer bowl and add more water below the bowl.
2. In the bowl, put the carrots and beet parts, then bring them to a boil.
3. Lower the heat to medium-low for 10 minutes, cover the pot until the carrots and beets are tender.
4. In a blender, mix all ingredients and blend until smooth.

5. Move the paste to a medium bowl, bring it to a boil, and then simmer for 20 minutes at the medium-low level.

Rhubarb Chutney

Cooking Time: 15 minutes

Serving Size: 4

Calories: 34.7

Ingredients:

- ¼ cup honey
- 1 lb. rhubarb, sliced
- ½ cup chopped onion
- ½ teaspoon cloves
- ½ teaspoon black pepper
- 1 teaspoon cumin
- ½ teaspoon cinnamon
- ¼ cup apple cider vinegar
- ½ tablespoon grated fresh ginger
- 1 large garlic clove

Method:

1. Put the first ingredients into a medium saucepan.
2. Turn the heat to medium-high, then whisk until mixed.
3. Remove the rhubarb, raisins, and onions, and stir again.
4. Cook until the rhubarb begins to melt and the sauce thickens.

Onion and Bacon Jam

Cooking Time: 20 minutes

Serving Size: 2

Calories: 40

Ingredients:

- Fresh crack black pepper
- ¼ cup coconut amino

- 1 tablespoon fresh thyme
- 2 pieces of thick-cut pastured bacon
- 1 ½ lb. Vidalia onions (sliced)
- Celtic sea salt, to taste

Method:

1. Heat a Dutch oven over medium-high heat and prepare the bacon until it is thoroughly cooked.
2. Remove the bacon and clean it on a paper towel.
3. Cook the chopped onion over the moderate flame in the oven, stirring regularly, for around 45 minutes or until browned and caramelized.
4. Cut the bacon and add it to the onion.
5. Mix the amino acids, thyme, and black pepper to the coconut.
6. Cook for the next 10 minutes or until the jam is heavy and thoroughly caramelized (often stirring).
7. Serve over chopped cucumbers, vegetables, grilled beef, or paleo carrot sticks to cool and serve.

Garlic Mayo

Cooking Time: 15 minutes

Serving Size: 4

Calories: 121

Ingredients:

- ¼ teaspoon salt
- ½ cup warm filtered water
- ¼ cup olive oil
- ½ cup coconut concentrate (slightly warmed)
- 4 cloves garlic

Method:

1. Place the coconut extract, hot water, olive oil, garlic powder, and salt in a blender to produce the mayo.

2. Mix on high until the mixture thickens for a minute or two.
3. Alternatively, you can put it in the fridge for twenty minutes or cool at ambient temperature for an hour.
4. Thin the mixture with water until the desired consistency is obtained, if you choose to put it in a cold bowl.

Blueberry Coconut Butter

Cooking Time: 10 minutes

Serving Size: 5

Calories: 136

Ingredients:

- 2 packages of (unsweetened shredded) coconut
- 3 tablespoons honey
- 3 cups fresh blueberries
- ¼ cup of coconut oil
- ¼ cup lemon juice (fresh squeezed)

Method:

1. Transform the processed coconut on medium speed using a high-speed blender until it changes into butter.
2. Use the tamper to carefully force the coconut down through the blender's blades when crushing it; this will take less than a minute to start this process.
3. Blend in the specified coconut oil, lime juice, and flavoring.
4. Using the tamper to drive the blueberries downwards into the blades, add the blueberries to the food processor and blend on fast until smooth.
5. Divide the Blueberry Coconut Butter into five glass preservation jars, leaving at the top of each container an inch of space.

6. Within a week, refrigerate to consume; preserve the remainder to maintain freshness.

Basil Pesto

Cooking Time: 5 minutes

Serving Size: ½ cup

Calories: 81.6

Ingredients:

- ½ teaspoon of sea salt
- 6 cloves organic garlic
- ¼ to ½ cup olive oil
- 4 ounces organic basil
- 3 teaspoon nutritional yeast

Method:

1. In a food processor, pulse the basil, healthy yeast, ginger, garlic, and salt until the basil leaves are roughly diced.
2. Stream in the olive oil gradually and continue to blend until the pesto is creamy.
3. In a Mason jar, refrigerate or freeze.

Avocado Cream Sauce

Cooking Time: 5 minutes

Serving Size: 4

Calories: 109

Ingredients:

- 2 tablespoons olive oil
- 1 tablespoon fresh lemon juice
- ½ teaspoon ground black pepper
- 3 cloves garlic (minced)
- 2 large avocados (peeled and pit removed)
- ¼ cup packed fresh basil leaves
- ½ teaspoon of sea salt

Method:

1. In a food processor, put all of the sauce components and blend for 15 seconds or until creamy.
2. If needed, check and add additional salt and black pepper.

AIP Carrot Ginger Sauce

Cooking Time: 20 minutes

Serving Size: 5

Calories:

Ingredients:

- 1 teaspoon of fresh ginger (peeled and minced)
- 1 teaspoon of salt
- 1 teaspoon of honey
- 2 tablespoons of (chopped) green onions
- 2 teaspoon of apple cider vinegar
- ¼ cup of grated carrot
- 3 tablespoon of fresh orange juice

Method:

1. In a food processor, put all of the sauce components and blend for 15 seconds or until creamy.
2. If needed, check and add additional salt and black pepper.

Teriyaki Sauce

Cooking Time: 10 minutes

Serving Size: 4

Calories: 76

Ingredients:

- ½ tablespoon arrowroot starch
- 1 tablespoon water
- ¼ teaspoon ginger powder
- ¾ cup coconut amino
- 1 teaspoon garlic powder
- 1 teaspoon onion powder
- ½ teaspoon Blackstrap molasses
- 2 tablespoon honey

Method:

1. In a shallow bowl, combine the arrowroot with the water.
2. In a cup, add the remaining ingredients and mix. Then add and whisk in the arrowroot combination.
3. Through a shallow saucepan, add the mixture and set over low heat. Simmer until it thickens.
4. Let it cool and keep for up to four days in the refrigerator in a glass pan. Until eating, reheat over low pressure.

Nightshade-Free Cherry BBQ Sauce

Cooking Time: 35 minutes

Serving Size: 3 cups

Calories: 69

Ingredients:

- ¼ cup vinegar
- 1 teaspoon sea salt
- 3 cups cherries
- ¼ cup maple syrup
- 5 cloves garlic
- 3 tablespoons coconut oil
- 1 large yellow onion

Method:

1. On medium-high heat, heat the coconut oil in a frying pan.
2. Add the onion when it's prepared, and fry for 10 minutes until its golden brown.
3. Add the garlic and roast, tossing, until fragrant, for another couple of minutes.
4. Add the cherries, syrup, vinegar, and sea salt.
5. Cook for twenty minutes, uncovered, or until the paste thickens substantially.
6. Switch to a blender and blend until thoroughly mixed to a high degree.

Conclusion

The AIP diet is an exclusion diet intended for those with an autoimmune disease to reduce symptoms. The first step of the diet excludes many kinds of foods that can induce inflammation and result in leaky gut. Slowly, foods are first reintroduced and tested for tolerance. The AIP diet is a stricter version of the Paleo diet, and on the AIP diet, certain foods that are included on the Paleo diet, such as nuts, beans, eggs, and dairy products, are gradually omitted. While this diet can help alleviate symptoms for those with an autoimmune disease, it should be combined with other safe changes in lifestyle to achieve the best outcomes.

It may also feel like your signs of disease and well-being are out of your hands when your immune system assaults itself after you struggle with an autoimmune disease. Although every day, there are several things you can do that can help promote your recovery and general well-being. Based on each specific person and their particular illness, the right autoimmune disorder diet and lifestyle will differ. But it can be beneficial for certain people to use traditional techniques, such as reducing weight, handling stress, prioritizing proper sleep, consuming anti-inflammatory diets, avoiding gluten, and improving the intestinal microbiota.

Give the methods described in this book a go, and then see how your health condition affected by the disease will improve gradually. With a few quick improvements to your everyday routines, you might be able to feel some relief from your symptoms. If you are searching for a different and effective diet and lifestyle support with autoimmune disorders, in that case, this book offers comprehensive details on the health of the body with diet plan, lifestyle choices, and delicious recipes.